Contents

My Healing Journey

~~Untitled Introduction~~

Katherine Anne (Rose) Hunt

April 28, 2011 – Thursday Eve

Before Treatment Begins

The Beginning

As you begin this medical journey, what lies heavily on your mind?

CFS - Chronic Fatigue Syndrome
I am always so very tired.
My body aches & is so very stiff.
My memory especially short-term,
is a challenge. I am always checking
myself for facts & remembering the past.
My eyesight is challenging. Many times
I find myself trying to read grocery
labels & signs. Arthritis is taking
over my joints. I try to ignore
symptoms when they appear. Life
just happens: Age is a reality!!
My goal is to minimize attention to
my pain. Pacing myself helps.

"Don't be ashamed to say what you are not ashamed to think."

— *Michel de Montaigne*

Recommendations

You decide, along with your caregiving team, which treatments to undergo, so it is very important that you understand your treatment options.

What do you think about the recommendations? What does your instinct tell you about each course of treatment?

What do family members and friends think about your doctor's recommendations?

"Trust that still, small voice that says, 'This might work and I'll try it.'"

— *Diane Mariechild*

Your Treatment Decision

Which course of action will you take? What are your reasons?

Will you be able to look back on this decision and remember why you made it?

How do the important people in your life feel about your decision? If they disagree, can you let it be okay that they have their opinions, knowing that the decision is yours to make?

_____

_____

_____

_____

_____

_____

_____

_____

_____

_____

_____

_____

"No trumpets sound when the important decisions of our life are made.

Destiny is made known silently." — *Agnes de Mille*

Your Hopes and Fears

Before treatment starts could be your most fearful time.

Search your mind and your heart. What do you think will happen?

What do you hope will happen? What pain (physical and emotional) do you fear? Do you know yet how the pain can be managed?

Writing down your fears may lessen their effect on you.

_____

_____

_____

_____

_____

_____

_____

_____

_____

_____

_____

_____

_____

"There is no medicine like hope, no incentive so great, and no tonic so powerful as expectation of something tomorrow." — *O. S. Marden*

Taking Stock

Before treatment begins, take stock of yourself mentally, emotionally, spiritually, socially, financially, physically and sexually.

Is there anything you need to do or say or arrange?

"To be at peace with ourselves, we need to know ourselves."

— *Caitlin Matthews*

Recurrence

If this is a recurrence of a previous cancer, or the occurrence of an additional type of cancer, how are you dealing with it?

What similar thoughts and feelings are you having this time?

What different thoughts and feelings are you having?

What did you learn before that can help you through this journey?

_____

_____

_____

_____

_____

_____

_____

_____

_____

_____

_____

_____

_____

"I have learned to use the word 'impossible' with the greatest caution."

— *Werner von Braun*

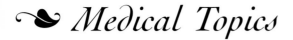 *Medical Topics*

Diagnosis

What type of cancer do you have?

How did you feel when you heard the diagnosis?

Was anyone with you when you found out?

"When I was told I had cancer I was very scared because I heard from TV,
the radio and my Mom and Dad that cancer was a serious disease.

But there was nothing I could do about it but wait to get it over with."

— *Betty, age 9*

Additional Input

You may feel a sense of urgency to get the cancer out of you; however, this is the time to gather information about your type of cancer and to learn about all options available to you.

What have you learned from other sources, such as the Internet, a second opinion, books, family members or friends who have had your type of cancer, the American Cancer Society, alternative healing practitioners, etc.?

"Look and you will find it — what is unsought will go undetected."

— *Sophocles*

Your [redacted] Doctor

Your oncology doctor, or medical oncologist, will be an important constant in your life, both during treatments and at checkups in years to come. Is this someone you feel comfortable with?

Can you ask candid questions and speak your mind with this person? Does your doctor answer your questions to your satisfaction?

"What we need is more people who specialize in the impossible."

— *Theodore Roethke*

Before ▬▬▬▬

What has your surgeon told you about this procedure?

Do you have any remaining questions that you need to ask?

_____

_____

_____

_____

_____

_____

_____

_____

_____

_____

_____

_____

"To gain that which is worth having, it may be necessary to lose everything else." — *Bernadette Devlin*

❧ About

Who are the people who manage your chemotherapy?

How do you feel toward them?

How do they treat you?

_____

_____

_____

_____

_____

_____

_____

_____

_____

_____

_____

_____

"There is no human relationship more intimate than that of nurse and

patient, one in which the essentials of character are more rawly revealed."
— *Dorothy Canfield*

Treatments

Describe the experience of having chemotherapy drugs enter and flow through your body.

Do you feel differently: Physically? Emotionally? Spiritually?

How do you spend your time while you are being treated?

_____

_____

_____

_____

_____

_____

_____

_____

_____

_____

_____

_____

"I knew who I was this morning but I think I've been changed several times since then." — *Alice, to the Caterpillar*

~~Chemotherapy~~ Side Effects

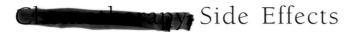

As you have more chemotherapy treatments, what do you notice?

What side effects have you experienced from chemotherapy?

What drugs or other remedies have you taken to combat the side effects? How have they worked?

_____

_____

_____

_____

_____

_____

_____

_____

_____

_____

_____

_____

_____

_____

"I've just gone through what is for me a huge personal crisis — losing my hair. I'm bald! I have to accept that the last four months have been

a horror for me and I did a good job coping with it, but now it shows!"
— *Carol J. Hinkley Thompson*

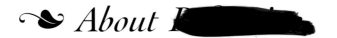

About ▮▮▮▮▮▮

Your ▮▮▮▮▮▮▮▮▮▮▮▮▮

Who are the people who manage your radiation?

How do you feel toward them?

How do they treat you?

_____

_____

_____

_____

_____

_____

_____

_____

_____

_____

_____

_____

"I took my children with me many times to watch the procedure.

They baked cookies to bring to the technicians." — *Christine Clifford*

▮▮▮▮▮▮Treatments

Describe the process of being radiated. Do you sense or imagine anything?

What goes through your mind as you are being treated?

How do you feel about having a tattoo on your skin?

_____

_____

_____

_____

_____

_____

_____

_____

_____

_____

_____

_____

_____

_____

"While lying in the big machine during radiation treatments,

I sang silently to myself, a devotional song to God." — *Priscilla Mueller*

~~Radiation~~ Side Effects

What do you notice as you have more radiation treatments?

Do you feel differently: Physically? Emotionally? Spiritually?

_____

_____

_____

_____

_____

_____

_____

_____

_____

_____

_____

_____

"What doesn't kill me makes me stronger."

— *Albert Camus*

❧ *More About Treatments*

After Surgery

What was the result of the surgery?

How has your body been changed surgically? How do you feel about those changes?

How do you think others perceive the changes?

_____

_____

_____

_____

_____

_____

_____

_____

_____

_____

_____

_____

"After my surgery, I was worried about all the things I wasn't going to be able to do. My Mom really helped me out on this.

'Don't look at the things you can't do, look at the things you can.'"
— *Kim, age 17*

Complementary Therapies

What are your thoughts about the different complementary therapies (e.g., acupuncture, guided imagery, nutritional changes, herbal remedies, energy healing, massage, art therapy, etc.)?

Can your doctor support your decision to explore these types of treatments?

Which complementary therapies are you participating in? Describe your experiences with them.

_____

_____

_____

_____

_____

_____

_____

_____

_____

_____

_____

_____

_____

"I went not only to the doctors, but also to barbers, bathkeepers, learned physicians, women, and magicians who pursue the art of healing;

I went to alchemists, monasteries, to nobles and the common folk, to the experts and the simple." — *Paracelsus*

Treatment Schedule

Describe the frequency and duration of your cancer treatments.
Is there a rhythm or pattern to them?

How do you feel if your treatment has to be postponed or the
dosage changed?

we are challenged to change ourselves." — *Victor Frankel*

Preconceived Notions

What preconceived notions did you have about cancer?

What preconceived notions did you have about chemotherapy or radiation?

What do you know now that you didn't know before you were diagnosed?

_____

_____

_____

_____

_____

_____

_____

_____

_____

_____

_____

_____

"It's what you learn after you know it all that counts."

— *John Wooden*

Hospital Visits

What goes through your mind when you go to the hospital? When you leave the hospital?

If someone takes you, what do you talk about?

Do you interact with other cancer patients?

_____

_____

_____

_____

_____

_____

_____

_____

_____

_____

_____

_____

"We did not all come over on the same ship,

but we are all in the same boat." — *Bernard Baruch*

As Treatments Progress

Write about the weariness you feel as treatments continue. Can you compare it to anything?

Can you find a new way to think about your treatments, e.g., pretend chemotherapy is a part-time job you go to, radiation is a vacation day from work, etc.?

What recurring thoughts have you had about your treatments or about anything?

_____

_____

_____

_____

_____

_____

_____

_____

_____

_____

_____

"Out of suffering have emerged the strongest souls;

the most massive characters are seared with scars." — *E. H. Chapin*

Final Treatments

What do you think about as you finish your treatments?

How do you feel about the medical staff who have treated you?

_____

_____

_____

_____

_____

_____

_____

_____

_____

_____

_____

"Better is the end of a thing than the beginning thereof.

— *Ecclesiastes 7:8*

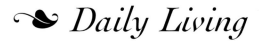

Daily Living

Routines

How do you spend your days?

Do you bathe differently? Do you have a wound to dress?

How much liquid do you drink? Does your diet keep changing? How are your bowels reacting?

"Success is the sum of small efforts, repeated day in and day out."

— *Robert Collier*

Rest

Does your body have different requirements for rest?

Do you sleep or dream differently?

Describe your bed. How do you feel about your bedroom or about your favorite couch?

_____

_____

_____

_____

_____

_____

_____

_____

_____

_____

_____

_____

"Rest is a good thing, but boredom is its brother."

— *Voltaire*

Money

What concerns do you have about money or insurance?

Do you have any worries about your ability to earn income?

Do you worry about your family managing without you?

_____

_____

_____

_____

_____

_____

_____

_____

_____

_____

_____

_____

"I got the bill for my surgery. Now I know what those doctors were wearing masks for." — *James H. Boren*

How has your sexuality been affected?

What worries do you have about fertility?

_____

_____

_____

_____

_____

_____

_____

_____

_____

_____

_____

_____

_____

_____

"The true joy of loving is an ecstasy of two bodies and souls mingling and uniting in poetry." — *Jolan Chang*

Upsets

What upsets you more than before?

What upsets you less?

Is there anything you miss in your life?

_____

_____

_____

_____

_____

_____

_____

_____

_____

_____

_____

_____

"And when it rains on your parade, look up rather than down.

Without the rain, there would be no rainbow." — *Jerry Chin*

Thinking and Learning

What sense do you make of why you got cancer?

Do you think the cause is genetic, environmental, karmic, random chance, or something else?

_____

_____

_____

_____

_____

_____

_____

_____

_____

_____

_____

"When an inner situation is not made conscious,

it appears outside as fate." — *C. G. Jung*

What Matters

What is more important than it used to be?

What is less important than it used to be?

Have you changed your mind about what is important in life? Why?

_____

_____

_____

_____

_____

_____

_____

_____

_____

_____

_____

_____

"When people say: she's got everything, I've only one answer:

I haven't had tomorrow." — *Elizabeth Taylor*

Benefits of Illness

What good things have you experienced from being ill?

_____

_____

_____

_____

_____

_____

_____

_____

_____

_____

_____

"Expect nothing; live frugally on surprise."

— *Alice Walker*

Writing

How do you like writing about your experience with cancer?

Do you ever feel like writing poetry?

Fill this page and the next with poetry or favorite sayings that you or others have written.

_____

_____

_____

_____

_____

_____

_____

_____

_____

_____

_____

_____

_____

"Writing, which is my form of celebration and prayer,

is also my form of inquiry." — *Diane Ackerman*

Loose Ends

What loose ends need tidying up?

What feels incomplete in your life?

What do you need to say to people to feel complete?

What do you need to accomplish?

_____

_____

_____

_____

_____

_____

_____

_____

_____

_____

_____

_____

_____

"You must do the thing you think you cannot do."

— *Eleanor Roosevelt*

Thoughts of Mortality

What thoughts have you had about your funeral, memorial service or obituary?

What do you want it to say on your gravestone?

Is your will current? Does it say what you want it to say?

What empty spaces would your death leave?

_____

_____

_____

_____

_____

_____

_____

_____

_____

_____

_____

_____

_____

_____

_____

"My days are swifter than a weaver's shuttle."

— *Job 7:6*

Learning

What are you learning about yourself?

What are you learning about others?

What are you learning about what it means to be human?

"There are some things you learn best in calm, and some in storm."

— *Willa Cather*

❧ *People in Your Life*

Circle of Support

On whom can you depend to support you, listen to you, drive you to appointments?

Describe your relationship with each person.

_____

_____

_____

_____

_____

_____

_____

_____

_____

_____

_____

_____

_____

_____

"Some people go to priests; others to poetry; I to my friends."

— *Virginia Woolf*

Support Groups

A cancer patient support group is a place where you can express your fears and desires and be understood by others in a similar situation. You may join at any time.

What are your thoughts and feelings about joining a support group?

What would be helpful about sharing your experience with other cancer patients?

What would be helpful about others sharing their experience with you?

_____

_____

_____

_____

_____

_____

_____

_____

_____

_____

_____

"Finding the right support group is like buying a new pair of shoes.

You may have to try on a few before you find the right fit."
— *Susan Sturges Hyde*

Your Family

How do you think your illness is affecting your siblings, parents or other family members?

Do you interact differently with anyone?

Does anyone treat you differently?

_____

_____

_____

_____

_____

_____

_____

_____

_____

_____

_____

_____

_____

"We live in others, and they in us."

— *Sigmund Freud*

Your Children

What are your thoughts and feelings about your children in regard
to your cancer?

How have they reacted to you, your illness and your treatments?

_____

_____

_____

_____

_____

_____

_____

_____

_____

_____

_____

_____

_____

"Out of your vulnerabilities will come your strength."

— *Sigmund Freud*

Reactions from Friends, Coworkers and Strangers

How do you think your illness is affecting your closest friends?

Are you surprised at how any of your friends have reacted to your cancer? Who has stayed away? Who has shown up unexpectedly?

How do people react to you when they learn about your illness? How do you feel about their reactions?

_____

_____

_____

_____

_____

_____

_____

_____

_____

_____

_____

_____

"A real friend is one who walks in when the rest of the world walks out."

— *Walter Winchell*

Gifts and Cards

Have you received any gifts or cards?

Which are your favorites? Why?

List the senders and what they sent or gave you.

"What we get on our birthday is a present. A gift comes unexpected and without wrapping paper, like a smile." — *Barry Neil Kaufman*

Appreciation

Who has been especially kind to you?

On your good days, do you call or send thank-you notes
to people who have been thoughtful?

"No duty is more urgent than that of returning thanks."

— *Saint Ambrose*

Helping Others

People often feel better when they reach out to help others.

Who might benefit from your presence, advice, a kiss on the cheek or a shoulder to cry on?

_____

_____

_____

_____

_____

_____

_____

_____

_____

_____

_____

"My chemo nurse said, 'You are strong. You will be able
to help other people go through this someday.'

She was right. A year later I helped a friend go through hers."

— *Priscilla Mueller*

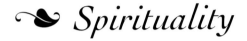 *Spirituality*

Spiritual Comfort

What prayers, hymns, music, affirmations or other spiritual practices give you comfort?

What parts of the bible or other religious or spiritual books soothe you?

Write the words here.

"I'm for anything that gets you through the night, be it booze or religion."

— Frank Sinatra

Higher Power

Has your relationship with God or a higher power changed?

Do you feel a need to reconnect with a place of worship?

Do you pray? What do you pray for?

Write your prayers here.

_____

_____

_____

_____

_____

_____

_____

_____

_____

_____

_____

_____

"Prayer is an exercise of the spirit, as thought is of the mind."

— Mary F. Smith

Clergy

Have you spoken with a member of the clergy? What did you talk about?

_____

_____

_____

_____

_____

_____

_____

_____

_____

_____

_____

"Faith is not belief. Belief is passive. Faith is active."

— *Edith Hamilton*

Laughter

When was the last time you laughed?

How do others react to your joking?

Do you appreciate gallows humor?

"Tell people that you are not dead yet and you want to laugh until your last breath." — *Patty Wooten*

Like a Child

How are you like a child?

What comforts from childhood still calm you?

Do you take a stuffed animal to bed?

_____

_____

_____

_____

_____

_____

_____

_____

_____

_____

_____

_____

_____

"One of the most obvious facts about grownups to a child is that

they have forgotten what it is like to be a child." — *Randall Jarrell*

Pets

What does the presence of your pet mean to you now?

Do you talk to your pet?

How has your pet been a pal?

"Until one has loved an animal, a part of one's soul remains unawakened."

— *Anatole France*

Happiness

Look out the window. Look in your bookcase. Look around the dinner table. Look everywhere.

List 10 things that make you happy. Then list 10 more. Fill the pages.

_____

_____

_____

_____

_____

_____

_____

_____

_____

_____

_____

_____

"Gloom we have always with us, a rank and sturdy weed,

but joy requires tending." — *Barbara Holland*

Insights and Miracles

What epiphanies or miracles have been manifested since your
treatment began?

_____

_____

_____

_____

_____

_____

_____

_____

_____

_____

_____

_____

"There are only two ways to live your life. One is as though

nothing is a miracle. The other is as though everything is a miracle."
— *Albert Einstein*

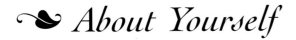 *About Yourself*

Nurturing Yourself

List the ways you comfort or nurture yourself.

What rituals give you comfort?

"I never loved another person the way I loved myself."

— *Mae West*

Loss of Dignity

What indignities have you had to put up with at the hospital?

How do you feel when that happens?

How do you think others around you feel?

"There are so many indignities to being sick and helpless. . . ."

— *Anna Roosevelt Halsted*

Control

What do you think you have control over?

What do you think you don't have control over?

What do you want to have happen that is beyond your control?

_____

_____

_____

_____

_____

_____

_____

_____

_____

_____

_____

_____

_____

"I need to take an emotional breath, step back, and remind myself who's actually in charge of my life." — *Judith M. Knowlton*

Your Appearance

How has your appearance changed?

How do your clothes feel on you? How much weight have you lost
or gained?

If your hair fell out, what do you want it to look like when it
grows back?

"Even I don't wake up looking like Cindy Crawford."

— *Cindy Crawford*

Photos

How do you feel about photos of yourself during this period in
your life?

Use these pages as a gallery to paste photos or drawings of you:
from before you got sick, during your treatments, as you get better.

"All photographs are there to remind us of what we forget."

— *John Berger*

Goals

What promises have you made to yourself? If you beat this disease
you'll _____?

What goals or milestones do you look forward to (e.g., wedding,
birth, vacation, etc.)?

_____

_____

_____

_____

_____

_____

_____

_____

_____

_____

_____

_____

"Promises are the uniquely human way of ordering the future."

— *Hannah Arendt*

Image

What or whom do you see in the mirror?

Do you detect a change in your presence? Has your sense of yourself changed?

_____

_____

_____

_____

_____

_____

_____

_____

_____

_____

_____

_____

_____

"I look in the mirror through the eyes of the child that was me."

— *Judy Collins*

Counseling

There are social workers, psychotherapists, chaplains and other professionals who specialize in helping cancer patients examine deep-seated thoughts and fears.

Have you spoken with a counselor? What did you discuss? How did you feel afterward?

If you are troubled but have not sought out a counselor, what's holding you back?

_____

_____

_____

_____

_____

_____

_____

_____

_____

_____

_____

_____

"Is it sufficient that you have learned to drive the car, or shall we look and see what is under the hood?

Most people go through life without ever knowing." — *June Singer*

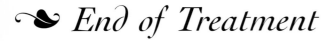 # *End of Treatment*

Prognosis

What prognosis has your doctor given after all your treatments?

What will you be able to do that was off limits to you during treatment?

How do you feel about being done with the treatments?

———————————————————————————

———————————————————————————

———————————————————————————

———————————————————————————

———————————————————————————

———————————————————————————

———————————————————————————

———————————————————————————

———————————————————————————

———————————————————————————

———————————————————————————

———————————————————————————

"Live each day as if it were the last day of your life,

because so far, it is." — *Unknown*

Fear of Recurrence

Explore your feelings about the possibility of cancer recurring in your body.

What message would a recurrence hold for you?

How do you think you would deal with a recurrence?

Do you foresee a day when you will not think about cancer?

_____

_____

_____

_____

_____

_____

_____

_____

_____

_____

_____

"It's not whether you get knocked down, it's whether you get up."

— *Vince Lombardi*

Leaving the Cocoon

When they have successfully completed their treatments and their regular appointments stop, some people feel they emerge from a protective aura, or cocoon, of care.

How do you feel about leaving what has become familiar to you?

"A ship in harbor is safe, but that is not what ships are built for."

— *John A. Shedd*

Thanking Your Caregivers

How could you show your thanks to your treatment team?

How could you show your thanks to the other caregivers in your life?

"Big-heartedness is the most essential virtue on the spiritual journey."

— *Matthew Fox*

Looking Back

What have you learned from this experience?

How have you changed?

What or who has meant the most to you?

What could you say to someone who has just been diagnosed with your type of cancer?

_____

_____

_____

_____

_____

_____

_____

_____

_____

_____

_____

_____

_____

"In the depths of winter I finally learned there was in me

an invincible summer." — *Albert Camus*

Your Future

Grandma Moses said, "If I didn't start painting, I would have raised chickens."

What would you have done if you hadn't been diagnosed with cancer?

What will you do when you recover?

What have you always wanted to do but have never had the nerve to try?

_____

_____

_____

_____

_____

_____

_____

_____

_____

_____

_____

_____

"We must be willing to get rid of the life we've planned,

so as to have the life that is waiting for us." — *Joseph Campbell*

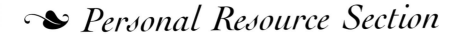 *Personal Resource Section*

Questions to Ask

What do you want to ask your medical team?

Record your questions here and take this journal with you to your medical appointments so you can write down the answers.

Test Results

Use these pages to keep track of your medical tests, including your white and red blood cell and platelet counts. Use the Comments column to record your doctors' comments and your own.

DATE	TEST	RESULTS	COMMENTS

DATE	TEST	RESULTS	COMMENTS

DATE	TEST	RESULTS	COMMENTS

DATE	TEST	RESULTS	COMMENTS

Contacts

Keep a central list of names and phone numbers of all the people on
your care team — medical oncologist, radiation oncologist, primary
care physician, chemo nurses, radiation technicians, pharmacist, clergy,
social worker, psychologist, complementary treatment practitioners,
nutritionist, drivers, meal preparers, babysitters, and so on.

NAME   **PHONE**

NAME   **PHONE**

NAME	PHONE

NAME   PHONE

Important Dates

Write or paste your treatment schedule here. It is wise to write in pencil in case your treatment dates change.

❧ *Author's Note*

I would appreciate your feedback about this journal: how it has helped you, additional topics and prompting questions that would be helpful, your own inspirational quotes, where others could learn about this journal. Please send your comments to:

Margie Davis
The Healing Way
c/o Element Books, Inc.
160 North Washington Street
4th Floor
Boston, MA 02114 USA
or email: margie@writingtoheal.com

Best wishes for good health.